Flat Tummy Secrets

Everything You Need to Know to Lose Weight Naturally and Effectively

Tammy Thomas

Copyright

Terms of Use

Any information provided in this book is through the author's interpretation. The author has done strenuous work to reassure the accuracy of this subject. If you wish you attempt any of the practices provided in this book, you are doing so with your own responsibility. The author will not be held accountable for any misinterpretations or misrepresentations of the information provided here.

All information provided is done so with every effort to represent the subject, but does not guarantee that your life will change. The author shall not be held liable for any direct or indirect damages that result from reading this book.

Contents

Introduction

Well, let's face it. We all hate having to go through the effort of losing weight. It's a lot harder to lose than to gain, that's a fact.

In addition to that, when we are in the process of losing weight, we are very limited as to what type of food we can eat. Of course, healthy food is a given and is will make us healthy eaters. Junk food, on the other hand, will only harm your body. We all know this but we prefer junk food over healthy food anyways. That's the way many people work.

Now, what sets those who are trying to lose weight and those who only have to maintain their weight is the fact that the maintainers are those who can better control themselves and their eating habits.

Let's be honest here, for those who has never attempted to lose weight before will not know where to start. Even if you do, you most likely won't know the proper way to do it without wanting to give up in the long run or to have to brutally torture your body with hunger and stress.

The truth is, dieting is a very simple process. It might take some effort and willpower here and there, but it's not something that you'll have to constantly force yourself to do. Eventually, if you don't think about it, it'll turn into a habit, especially if you're going to follow the methods used in this book.

Did You Know

Let's get started on the facts before we head towards the learning part of the book.

Did you know that everything that you have been told about losing weight is wrong?

That's not very unexpected considering the fact that many people in society would rather lose weight quickly rather than slowly.

This is where the media steps in and starts to throw out lies in order to feed your brain. Obviously, when you're hungry you would eat. Likewise, your brain does the same thing. It's hungry for knowledge and it's going to swallow the first information that it finds whether the information is correct or not.

Did you also know that there is a 95% failure rate for those who have attempted to go on a diet? That means that only 5% passes which is pretty sad considering the fact that the failure rate is so high. This is because those in the failure rate are either doing something wrong or they just no longer have the motivation to continue.

We all know that losing weight is a pain, but there are way too many people giving up too quickly.

Unfortunately, out of the whole U.S. population, 67% of the population is either obese or overweight.

When you're considering about going on a diet, it's best to research different methods. Don't go by what the media tell you. Chances are they're lying. You've seen it all the time: weight loss shows, weight loss pills, and weight loss foods.

Let's be realistic here. Almost anything that you see on TV is false and that whoever makes them is trying to empty your wallet for their own benefit. I'm not saying that you shouldn't watch TV, just don't believe every single word you hear when watching.

Consider some failed methods: starving, eating low-fat food, and taking diet pills. None of these works. For one reason, starving isn't even a healthy diet plan. Not only are you going to damage your body, but you'll also be easily vulnerable to stress and depression. There's also anorexia if you manage to make it that far.

Secondly, eating low-fat food is only going to make you fatter. I'll get to this explanation later on.

Thirdly, diet pills. Those might work but don't count on it ever lasting. Diet pills are like fairy dust. It's fake and only works on movies. Don't ever bother starving yourself either. That's also going to backfire for many purposes.

I'll tell you something truthful that you won't believe: fat helps you lose weight. Don't think that it's a load of bull. It's true. This is because fat helps you lose weight by filling you up and keeping your hunger satisfied. The point of low-fat is to keep your stomach unsatisfied. When your stomach is satisfied, you won't have the urge to eat more.

Besides, your body needs fat in order to burn off the other fats. It sounds surreal but that's the way it goes. However, that doesn't mean that you should allow yourself to eat any type of fat food.

Fats may be good to consume but you have to know which one to consume. There are bad fats and good fats which you will learn more of later on.

So you've often heard about how carbs are the source of what makes you fat. Well, that's not the case. Carbs doesn't really do much. Likewise, it's not the carbs but the calories that accompanies it.

If there is a low carb amount in your diet, you'll most likely get sick. Even so, not all carbs are equal. You should keep that in mind.

The best advice you can ever get about losing weight is to eat wisely. Weight loss isn't around complexity but simplicity. It's a given that if weight loss was too hard a process then no one would continue doing it.

More or less, no one would want to continue doing it. The simpler weight loss is, the easier it is to succeed. Because it'll be easier to succeed, we'll be more incline to finishing it and not giving up half way in.

Did you also know that being able to stay slim and being healthy does not mean that you are going on a diet. Those ideas may seem similar but they're really not.

It actually varies on how you live your life. Staying slim is to maintain your current weight. Being healthy is to live and eat healthy food.

Dieting is the process of losing weight. You see, they are similar but also different.

Here is the big shock about weight loss: stop trying to lose weight. If you always have weight loss in your mind, it's going to be troublesome in the long run. It's good to focus on it, but as time goes on, it's going to develop into a routine.

The secret is to not think about it too much. Just do it and you'll be used to it.

Slow and Steady

We've all heard of the saying "Slow and steady wins the race." Well weight loss is the same thing. If you slowly work at decreasing your weight, you'll have an easier time losing weight.

The main reason why most people aren't losing weight is because they're trying to lose weight too quickly. Even if you did succeed in losing weight at a fast rate, all that weight that you've lost is going to come back.

Once it comes back, it's going to be twice as hard to lose it compared to the first time. In addition to that, losing weight too quickly is going to damage your body. This is because you're probably going through a harsh method that takes a lot of will power to accomplish.

Believe it or not, there are actually side effects to losing weight too quickly. It's not as if the side effects are good anyways.

A good pace to lose weight is to lose only 1-2 pounds per week. That may seem little but it'll add up. Losing weight depends more on time rather than effort. It's not something that you should only spend a month or two on.

If you were thinking about losing about 30 pounds or more in a month, give up now. For one thing, it's going to require a huge amount of effort and willpower from you. It's not going to be easy. In the end, it's not going to be surprising if you break down in the long run.

Hardly anyone can achieve that goal but there have been many people trying to achieve it. You should at least get a minimum of 1,600 calories per day. If you go under that, your body is going to conserve every calorie to eat rather than burning off the calories that you already have.

In doing so, it's going to result to you gaining the weight that you wanted to lose. This is because when your body is low on calories and fat, it goes on what is called "survival mode." Survival mode is basically a stage that your body has already established for you when you do not have enough food in your system. Your body isn't going to know that you chose not to eat. It's going to think that you're starving because you have nothing to eat.

It's common sense to know that no one can wake up one morning and instantly find that they're fat. It can work in movies through a magical spell caused by an evil witch or something but it's not going to work in reality. Even if there can be a magical force that tries to fatten you up over night, it'll most likely try to kill you rather than fatten you up. Just saying. Anyways, the only way for you to gain weight is through time.

If you are constantly eating unhealthy food, you may not realize it but it'll build up. If you're consuming more calories than you should per day then your weight is going to slowly build. You may think that a can of soda is harmless as of now because you're only taking it for one day. The next day you'll eat a bag of chips. The day after that you're eating donuts. All of these foods that you're eating per day is going to build up into something that would take weeks to lose.

In the end, you should take it slowly when you're trying to lose weight. Just like how weight can build up over time, losing it will take time.

Slow and steady is an easy way to lose weight and it also minimizes the risk of the weight ever coming back. It's also safe from a medical point of view seeing as you're not doing any tremendous damage to your body.

If you lose only 1-2 pounds per week it's not going to require much effort. You'll still be able to eat and stay full. You just have to make sure that whatever you're eating is healthy and doesn't go over the calories per day limit.

Myths

Nowadays, there seems to be myths of about almost anything. I'm actually not amazed about how there are myths about weight loss. I'll be honest; I actually believed some of these myths back when I didn't know any better. It's all about researching and finding the truth of the matter.

Most of these myths may seem correct but it's not. The point of myths is that it's not true but stated as if it were true. You'll most likely recognize most of them, if not all. Make sure you take note of them. These little rumors may seem harmless but once you start your weight loss routine, it can limit your ability to lose weight.

1. Starving

I like to call this myth the starving myth even if others may word it a little differently. Either way, the concept is the same. Basically, this is the myth where you would avoid meals in order to lose body fat. Well for one thing, you're going to actually gain the fat that you're trying so desperately to lose.

Secondly, you're going to start having cravings and hunger that is going to be very difficult for you to cope with. Eventually, you're going to get tired of coping with it and will eat something fattening.

Thirdly, you're going to damage your body and be vulnerable to stress. You might even get sick. That or you'll get anorexia.

Fourthly, you're going to fail. You won't even last. Just give up before you bother to try. I'm not saying this to challenge you. I'm saying this because it's not worth your time and effort.

2. Calories

Usually, most people would say that calories aren't important. Well, they are. I'd be lying to you if I also agreed that they weren't. Calories are actually very important. If you're planning on losing weight, pay close attention to them. They decide whether would you gain or lose weight. In order to lose weight, make sure that you don't consume more calories than what your body can burn off.

Though, keep in mind that consuming too little calories has the same effect as consuming too much. Make sure that you balance your calorie consumption properly. Also, don't buy low-fat products. They make you fatter. Eating low-fat food is like eating regular food minus the taste and plus the sugar. You're not getting much of a change through that method so don't waste your money.

3. Genes

Here is the popular one: fat genes. I used to be a short and overweight kid when I was little so I used to think that I had fat genes too because my mom would often tease me. Then I grew up and got taller. Now I'm just slightly chubby. To this day, I still think that it's because my body expanded. Anyways, that's beside the point.

The point is that fat genes do not exist. Fatness isn't hereditary. You can't really obtain fat through genes. Fat is just something that you gain on your own. If you're parents are overweight it might be possible that you would think that you've inherited that trait also, but it really isn't.

Obviously, when you're little, you would be easily influenced by what your parents do. If your parents are the type of eaters who will just eat anything they want at any time then you would most likely pick up that habit. That's the exact reason why you would also be overweight. You just end up picking up your parent's habits that's all. Nothing to it.

4. Diet Drinks

Isn't great that society nowadays have developed diet soda? You can totally drink as much as you want without having to worry about getting fat. Yeah right. Sorry to anyone who is a big fan of diet soda but drinking diet soda can kill you easier than actual soda. There is an actual research on it. On a side note, the truth is that diet soda uses a type of artificial sweetener called aspartame.

Aspartame is a chemical that is placed in diet soda drinks and the more diet sodas you have, the more you'll be craving for more sweets and sugar. When drinking diet soda you won't really gain weight like you do when you drink regular soda. However, that doesn't mean that the next thing you crave after that diet soda isn't going to be something fattening either. You're better off if you don't bother drinking any sodas at all.

5. Fat Free

Fat free foods work the same way as how diet sodas work. They contain the same amount of calories as the original product, if not more. So to all those people who were trying to lose weight by eating fat free foods, you're heading straight back to square one. There wasn't much progress you were making for yourself when you were eating fat free foods.

Technically, fat free foods weren't supposed to have a taste in the first place. However, if food doesn't have a taste to begin with, people would not buy them. Food companies realized this set back so they decided to replace the lack of taste with sugar. In the end, you're just eating something fattening without realizing it.

6. Metabolism

It's a common trait for those with slow metabolism to complain about those with fast metabolism. It's a lot easier for someone with a fast metabolism to lose weight compared to those with a slow metabolism. Nevertheless, did you know that metabolism is a flexible process?

Even if you have a slow metabolism, it can be boosted through exercise and physical activities. That's because the healthier you are the faster your metabolism is.

7. Exercise

Let's get this straight. You do need to diet even if you exercise a lot.

No matter how much you exercise, there is no way for you to be able to lose weight if you're constantly eating unhealthy foods. You don't even need to exercise if all you're doing is eating healthy foods. Understand that dieting would always win over exercise. The food that goes down your stomach has more effect on your weight compared to the amount of exercise that you do.

8. Walking

Because it's perfectly logical that walking does not do anything since walking is not even considered as an exercise. It's also perfectly logical as to why that above statement is wrong.

Walking is an exercise whether you disagree or not. Exercising is an activity that requires you to move your body in order to lose weight. Therefore, walking fits into this category. You may not realize it but if you're a heavy walker, you'd be able to burn off a good amount of calories without having to do any other heavy workout. You may think that walking doesn't necessarily do anything but it does and it can.

Obviously, walking isn't going to make any drastic change to your body in a short amount of time like other exercises, but it does something. Think about it. If you don't have the time or the money to go to the gym for a good workout, walking is a useful and easy exercise for burning weight. If you take a least 10,000 steps per day, you're actually burning off 250 calories per day. Also, taking 10,000 steps per day isn't difficult. That's only 2.5 miles

Weight Loss

Taking a step back, we've established the fact that losing weight is not just eating less and working out more. It requires an equal balance of both.

Here is the main reason why obesity is very high in the U.S. It's not that people don't know how to eat properly, but it's because they don't know when to stop eating or what to eat less of.

Back in the old days where food was still scarce, we didn't have enough to eat throughout the year. So, in response to that, our bodies kept storing fat in order to keep us alive from the lack of food. However, our bodies never actually set a limit as to how much fat we can store which is why obesity isn't a problem.

The more fat we stored in our bodies, the more energy we had available. This way, when we starve or lose weight, our bodies will start slowing down our metabolism in order to preserve the remaining amount of fat we have left.

Obviously, we don't have those issues nowadays. If we want food, we can go and buy it whenever we want.

There's an endless amount of food stores around every block. Unfortunately, our bodies are not aware of that. Don't attempting to starve yourself as a way to lose weight. Your body isn't going to think that you're doing it on purpose. In the end, your method is going to backfire.

Here's a fact: the faster you lose weight, the easier it is for you to regain weight. As I've stated before, if you cut down your food amount your body is going to turn down your metabolism. So when you start to eat again the fat will come back quickly since your metabolism is at its slowest performance.

The downfall is that, once those fats come back, it comes back in the form of pure fat. So, basically, you've just replaced your muscles with fat. That's not a very promising trade. I'm pretty sure you also agree with me. This is why you shouldn't try to lose weight too quickly.

Any method that allows you to lose weight at a fast rate isn't going to benefit you in the long run. It's typical that the American trend is to finish everything at a fast rate. However, for things like this, it's best if you just take it slow.

There are high health risks for those who try to lose weight too quickly. In addition, about 80% - 90% of people who has attempted weight loss regained all of their lost weight after 2 years.

For those who followed a low-calorie diet, like starving, regained more weight than the weight they lost. I've said this before: the more times you lose and regain weight, the harder it will be for you to lose it again.

So that means that your 2nd attempt to go on a diet will be more difficult than your first attempt.

I suppose now would be a good time to tell you about the risks of rapid weight loss: massive muscle loss, cardiac arrest, heat failure, kidney failure, anorexia and other eating disorders, lowered metabolism, nervousness, and depression. I'm pretty sure that all of these risks are as bad as the next one.

Hunger

There should be no reason as to why you would want to skip out on meals. Food is awesome. Honestly, I love food. If getting fat from eating wasn't an option I'd never stop eating. Besides, you can't defeat hunger.

Hunger is one of the strongest sensations a body can produce. In order to go against hunger you would need to have a strong amount of willpower and determination. Unfortunately, most people don't have that which makes the method of skipping meals impossible.

In weight loss, you are still able to eat enough meals a day without having to worry about gaining weight. Eating food with a high satiation per calories is one way to eat freely. This is because these types of foods will fill you up without giving you too much calories.

Remember that there are also good fats in food. Fats are what make you full from eating so it's only natural that you would need some in your food.

As I've stated, low-fat foods makes you want to eat more because it's filled with sugar. So stay on the safe side and eat regular food.

Protein is also good for the body as long as you don't have too much. You have to know how to balance the protein that you eat. If you don't have enough protein in your body, your blood sugar level will be all over the place.

Protein is what improves your body's ability to burn fat but that doesn't mean that you should take in too much of it. Be careful of how much you're taking in per day as you're eating.

Game

Everyone wants to win even if it's just a simple game. So, why not make weight loss a game? Just like a game, it'll have rules. Your opponents are unhealthy foods while your allies are healthy foods. If you keep eating unhealthy foods, you're losing to your opponents. It's going to sound wrong if I say that you'll win by eating your allies, but you get the point.

Make sure that you don't break any rules because, if you do, you'll be disqualified. You don't want to be kicked out of the game before you've even started now. That'll be embarrassing.

Even so, the rules aren't very difficult. As long as you follow them you'll be able to win the weight loss game.

1. Fooling yourself

Don't fool yourself. It'll be depressing if you do. In the weight loss game, you have nothing to be afraid about. No one is around to watch you or to criticize you. You're your own opponent. If you want to win then defeat yourself.

This is why you shouldn't bother wasting your time and effort playing this game if all you're going to do is fooling yourself of what you're doing. Be aware of your behavior and be careful of what you eat and how much you're eating.

It's fine if you wanted to pick up a back of chips and eat it because you're craving for it. It's not fine if you just end up saying, "I've already eaten something unhealthy so I'll continue tomorrow and eat what I want today." No. Eating one unhealthy snack and eating unhealthy for the rest of the day is two completely different things. Just because you eat something unhealthy for one meal time doesn't mean that it has to continue to the rest.

Also, don't make excuses to eat more or think that you aren't taking in that many calories. You probably are. Anything that you eat that is chemically made is going to contain a lot of calories. So stop lying to yourself. Don't be like other people who would fool themselves and make excuses for eating something that they weren't supposed to.

Everyone has cravings but that doesn't mean that you should push it. You can't just break away from your diet and continue onto the next day just because it's a new day. In dieting, every day counts and everything counts. You can't wing it. It's something that has to do with your body. You can't fool your own body so why bother.

2. Unfairness

Let's be honest, overweight people tend to look on the unfair side when looking at thin people. Whether or not you deny this is up to you. Regardless, it's true. However, it's not something that you should put yourself down for.

There's no such thing as unfairness when you're comparing your weight with someone else's. Everyone has had their fair share of having to lose weight at a certain point or having to maintain their weight even till today.

There are 3 types of thin people: those who are naturally thin, those who work to stay thin, and those who stay thin. Let's talk about why these types of people are so different from each other. For naturally thin people, they do not have to work hard to put off weight; however, they would need to work hard to put on weight. This is because the way their body works is different from anyone else. These types of people are very rare to find but you can see that they necessarily don't enjoy being thin all the time. It's not as if these people doesn't enjoy being thin but because they feel as it they are too thin compared to everyone else.

Moving to those who work to stay thin, these types of people have to work to maintain their weight. This is because they feel that it's necessary to stay thin. These are the types of people who are constantly watching what they eat and how much portions they eat per day. Thirdly, for those who stay thin, they don't necessarily have to work but they aren't exactly naturally thin either.

You can say that they're in the middle between the naturals and the hard workers. This is because these types of people only eat when they have to and exercise from time to time. They eat enough to fill them up for the day and they'll exercise whenever they feel like it.

There is nothing unfair about other people being thinner than you. Being thin is a choice. It's about health and feeling good. If you think that it's unfair for someone else to be thinner than you then those are your problem.

Your weight is the outcome of what you chose to eat. No one has anything to do with it. If you're really motivated into losing weight then you shouldn't whine about it. Just do it.

Set your priorities straight and everything else will fall into place. Eventually, whatever you do will turn into a habit.

3. Challenges

When you make up your mind to lose weight, you're setting yourself a challenge. If you don't have a plan to overcome that challenge then you won't be able to get anywhere. You'll be pushed back into square one before you're able to reach square two.

The best plan you can have is to make the fridge your friend. If you're like most people, the fridge would already be your friend. Well, give your fridge a higher standard than you did before because your fridge is what's going to affect your eating habit. If anything, always have a back up plan in case if your first plan failed. The more plans you have the better. The same applies with discouragement. Obviously, when you're attempting to lose weight, you're going to feel discourage from time to time. Even so, that's perfectly natural.

The best way to counteract this is to enter into the diet program with some mental toughness in mind. If you have the mentality of what to expect, it'll be 10 times easier for you to handle what's coming to you. This way you'll be expecting something bad to happen and you'll be thinking up ways to counter it. You won't lose motivation as easily if you're already predicting a brick wall to be in your way.

Another method is to take it slowly. You can't possibly do everything all at once. The best way is to do one thing at a time until you're used to it. Start with something easy and progress further once you feel comfortable doing it.

If you decide to take in everything at once, you'll eventually end up feeling powerless and stuck. You'll be making weight loss seem harder than it's supposed to be.

The whole of losing weight is that it's supposed to be easy for you. It's just gaining calories and losing it. You're probably thinking that it's easier said than done, but, honestly, it's easy regardless. It's just you that's making it hard.

4. Easy Way Out

You can't cheat when you're trying to lose weight. In an actual game, it might work if no one notices you doing it, but in weight loss you can't. That's because you're only cheating yourself and, obviously, you're going to pay. If you've ever bought weight loss pills, throw them out. I don't care if you paid a lot for it. It's not like you're getting anything worth while out of your money in the first place.

In the end, you've just got ripped off. You're not benefiting anything by using a pill that is chemically made. This might be reality but did you honestly believe in the fact that there was a weight loss pill to begin with? Did you actually believe that it's going to work without any side effects?

Think about it. It seems too good to be true simply because it is too good to be true. That's why you shouldn't take the easy way out. It's best if you just follow the natural way and eat healthy. At least you're doing something worth that's your money and the food that you're eating is going to help benefit you in many ways.

The simplest method is the one that produces the best results. So don't back away from it and take the easy route. You don't get through life by taking the easy route either. Even if you've hit a brick wall in the long run, don't give up.

Just keep going. Don't make it seem impossible for you to accomplish when it's not.

5. Unrealistic Goals

Whenever you're thinking about doing something, keep it realistic. Life isn't some fictional book that you're living. It's going to make your life a lot easier if you're realistic about a lot of things. Same thing applies for weight loss.

Like I said, if you try to lose weight too quickly, you're going to end up with a lot of frustration and headaches. That's going to stress you out even more and you're going to want to give up. I'm not going to be amazed if you do. It's pretty much expected.

When you make goals for yourself in terms of weight loss, balance it. Don't use a method that will help you lose weight too quickly and don't use a method that will take a long time for you to reach your goal.

Also, pick a goal that isn't too small and vague. That's like saying, "I'm going to lose 5 pounds this week," and that's all you say. Ok, we get that you want to lose 5 pounds. What of it? How are you going to lose 5 pounds? What are you going to do to achieve that goal? How are you going to do it? Answer these questions before establishing a goal.

The more precise you are the easier it will be for you to accomplish what you've set out for yourself. You won't change anything if you have a vague goal.

There are different types of goals for weight loss. You can set a goal stating that you will reach a certain weight by this certain date. An example would be 5 pounds in 2 weeks. If you want to be more precise, replace that 2 weeks with an exact date.

Once you've established that goal, plan how you'll accomplish it. Another goal would be what you would eat and what exercises you should do. So you'll plan what you'll eat and what you'll not eat for that certain amount of time and you'll plan what type of exercise you'd do and for how long you would do it.

The last goal would be how many pounds you would want to shed per week or month. This is a more relaxed goal depending on how much weight you would want to lose in that specific amount of time.

Despite the goals that you've established for yourself, make sure that you're committed to accomplishing it. It's ok if you're not 100% into it. No one is expecting your full effort.

If weight loss requires you to give your 100% effort all the time it wouldn't be easy anymore.

Remember, your determination decides the amount of effort that you're going to put into accomplishing your goals.

6. Sabotaging Thoughts

Every action begins with a thought. Even if you're acting on instincts there is some thought put in that. You're just thinking while doing compared to thinking before doing. That's the gist of it. Even so, when it comes to weight loss, most people tend to do things thinking that it'll be fine as long as they've ok'ed it for themselves. Sorry, but that isn't the case. If you let yourself use a faulty logic you won't be able to get anywhere with your goals.

You're just sabotaging yourself in the end. No one is going to be around to say no to what you do when you're alone. It's up to you to be sincere with yourself.

Likewise, if you were to fail don't give up for the rest of the day. If you make a mistake and give in to your cravings then that don't mean that you shouldn't continue making that mistake for the rest of the day. The point of a mistake is that you should fix it once you've done it. It's not going to benefit you in anyway if you continue making that mistake.

Setting Goals

As I was previously talking about goals, it's always good to make some preparations before you start your weight loss program.

In order to narrow down how strong your motivation is you need to make a list of the pros and cons of what you're getting yourself into before you start. It doesn't matter whichever side dominates in terms of reasons. It matters about which side is more important to you.

Of course, staying healthy should be your first and top choice so it would be difficult for me to understand if you chose the con over the pro. Anyhow, when you're getting yourself into the weight loss program, you're making a lifetime plan not a temporary diet goal.

Once you start there's no turning back which means that you would have to stick to your goal for a long time. If you're the type who can easily forget about something, write your goals down so you can remember it. Write it down, stick it somewhere, and look at it every day if that's the only way you'll be able to become motivated.

Remember, work small and then make your way up to the bigger goals. Don't do something difficult the moment you start. Start easy so you can last for a long time. Be realistic with your goals and the more specific they are the better. It'll be easier for you to accomplish them if they are.

Also, the best goals can be tracked for progress. This is because if you're easily able to keep track of what you've accomplished, you can give yourself feedback later on.

You'll be able to go back and correct your past mistakes and you can see what you can improve on for the future. Be sure to revise your goals every so often to fit your needs. After a while you're going to have to tweak it since there are things that have changed.

If you don't then you'll be stuck on the same square that you were last left on. Break down your goals in order to fit your needs. The speed of how fast you can finish your goals does not matter. The only thing that matters is how well you can accomplish them. Always plan ahead and plan daily for better results.

Keeping Track

Aside from setting your goals, it's always good to keep track of them for future purposes. When you're in the weight loss program, it's essentially helpful for you to keep track of what you eat.

Keeping a journal with you is the key to help you lose weight. It might seem tiring to constantly update yourself on what you eat, but you'll understand that it's going to become very useful when you've hit a wall.

By keeping track of your food consumptions, you can provide yourself with accurate data. It also provides clarity around habits and feelings, reminding you of your goals and motivates you as time goes on.

You should always try your best to keep your journal with you at all times, especially if you know that you're going to eat when you're away from home. If you have a big journal then it's expected and understandable that you wouldn't want to drag it everywhere with you since it's going to become a hassle.

What you can do is to carry those small, pocket-sized, mini-notebooks with you wherever you go. This way, it'll be a lot more convenient for you to carry the journal everywhere with you and you'll be able to transfer the data into your actual notebook whenever you have time. With this, nothing is lost and you'll always have the correct information provided when you look back on it.

When keeping track of data, make sure that you write it down immediately. Don't wait to write it down later thinking that you'll remember the exact amount of what you've eaten. Most likely, you won't. Once you're done immersing yourself in your food you won't be able to remember the amount of calories that you've eaten because you'll be distracted by other things.

It's good to trust yourself and it's good to have confidence in your memories, but it's bad if you don't know how to apply that confidence properly. If you want to be accurate then do it right away. No matter how well your memory is there's always a minor set back to it.

In weight loss, details are everything. Every number counts. This is because it is your body. Even the smallest amount of calories can add up into something bigger if you don't take careful note of it.

Usually, it's always the foods that contain the least amount of calories that we don't take note of. This is because we don't think that it affects us even if it does. If you take enough of each small amount then it'll accumulate into a higher amount.

I've mentioned this before. Don't lie to yourself. It's a pointless and futile effort. The only person you're cheating is yourself since no one else is sharing your body with you. When you write down the information in your journal the only person who is going to see it is you.

Unless if you're really planning on sharing it with someone, no one else has access to it besides you. With that being said, there's nothing that you should be embarrassed about. No one can really make fun of you if you've never showed it to them. Just be 100% honest with yourself.

Plateaus

Plateaus are the stage where you might start feeling that you're not making any progress or that you have stopped improving completely.

This is very common and expected for whatever you're doing. Nevertheless, there are 2 types of plateaus: mini-plateaus and the lengthy plateaus. Mini-plateaus don't do much harm.

It only lasts for 2-3 days or 2-3 weeks and it usually comes and goes. Throughout the weight loss process, you'll probably hit these mini-plateaus a few times before you're able to get use to them. It won't do much damage to your goals unless if you allow them to. Be careful though, if you go with the flow and let it drag on it's going to become the lengthy plateaus.

The lengthy plateau is the 2nd type of plateau. It can last beyond 3 weeks. These are the type of plateaus that you should watch out for because once you've hit them, it'll be hard to get out of. Usually, it'll take more effort for you to break apart from the lengthy plateaus since it's something that is caused by what you're doing to yourself, but if you manage to break from it, it means that you're ready to take a step forward and try something new.

There are a couple of ways to deal with plateaus. It's probably going to be useful, especially for the lengthy plateaus.

1. Calorie Consumption

For this method, it's good if you've been keeping a journal of your eating records. If you don't now is a good time to start one. Basically, whatever you eat will be recorded on that journal as well as the calories that it contains.

This way, it'll be easier for you to look back on it when you're in a pinch. It's ok if you guess the amount of calories you've eaten for that day, especially when you have to do some heavy calculations. Make sure that you count up all of the calories that you've eaten per day for the past week or so.

After you've done that you can check your records for consistency. If your records are inconsistent then that means that something is wrong. This would explain why you aren't making any progress in your weight loss or that you haven't been losing the weight that you wanted to lose.

If the records are fine, make sure that you aren't cheating yourself by eating something that you aren't recording. You're trying to solve the issue.

You should be careful when you're checking your records. If your records are inconsistent then look at the kind of foods you've been eating before making any changes. If there are certain foods that you're eating that holds more calories than the other foods then try switching it with something else. You can also try cutting back a couple of calories if the problem isn't necessarily caused by the foods that you're eating.

2. Reestablish

I've already mentioned this before; readjust your calorie consumption once every so often. Obviously, around this time, your body would most likely be changing and the amount of calories that you're consuming would also need to be readjusted to match that change.

If your body doesn't change then that means that you're doing something wrong. If that was the case then you have to readjust your methods and goals. Clearly, you're doing something wrong if nothing is different. Figure it out and change it into something better.

3. Change it up

When you're thinking of losing weight, you also have to take in the fact that exercise is a must. It doesn't matter how healthy you're eating or how well you're following the plan. You won't be able to easily lose the weight you want to lose if you're not bothering to exercise.

For those who already do exercise, it's best if you decide to change up your exercise routine if you already haven't done so. The thing about our bodies is that it can adapt very easily. If you're constantly doing the same exercise all the time then your body will adapt to it. This might be one reason why you're hitting a plateau.

You're probably doing the same type of routine every time you work out. If your only form of exercise is running then change it up once in a while. Stop running for a couple of days and try lifting weights in place of it. If you keep doing the same type of exercise all of the time then it will be harder for you to keep losing weight. If you feel conformable with the exercise that you're currently doing then the best way would be for you to pump up your workout. So if your regular workout is a 30 minutes jog per day then you should boost it up to one hour per day in order to burn off the calories that you had intended to burn.

If you don't want to upgrade then try another workout. You should be careful not to stay in the same work out for more than 5 weeks. That's usually the time it'll take for your body to adapt to the workout that you're doing. You should also try lifting weights if you haven't done so.

Losing weight is good but you can also gain some muscles along the way. I know that this type of exercise would be most men's first choice.

4. Break Away

This step should only be taken for a last resort. This is because it's the easiest method to do. All you have to do for this is to break away from your weight loss program.

It's natural that you'll get tired of sticking with the same weight loss program for a long time. Maybe your body has also gotten used to it for all you know. If the previous methods don't work, take a break from eating healthy and start eating whatever you want. Don't think about what you're consuming just eat to your heart's desire.

This will allow your body to reset your metabolism so you'll basically be resetting yourself back to stage one.

It's going to be expected that you'll gain some weight during this process but once you restart; however, your body won't hit the same plateau again. That doesn't mean that you'll stop hitting plateaus in general, it just means that you won't hit it at the exact same stage that you've hit it before.

You'll improve from it and the next time won't be as bad. The only thing that you have to remember from this method is that you cannot drag it out for a long time. Lengthy plateaus may last for more than 3 weeks but that doesn't mean that you can start eating whatever you want for more than 2-3 months. The longer you halt your weight loss program the harder it'll be for you to get back on track once you've restarted.

Maintenance

Believe it or not, it's a lot harder to maintain your weight rather than to lose it. This is because when you're losing weight, you have a strong determination to reach the goal that you've established for yourself.

Once you've accomplished that goal, is your next goal going to mean as much to you as the previous one? It should, but I wouldn't be amazed if it wasn't to some people. This is because you've already hit that weight that you want.

All you have to do now is to be careful to not to over eat and exercise what you eat off. You can end up eating unhealthy foods and still maintain a close number of the weight that you've gained just by exercising as long as you're careful of what you do.

At times like these, you should be someone who is very goal oriented. This is a good trait to have in life and it's going to help benefit you in the long run.

When you're goal oriented, you have a standard of your own and you stick with that standard. You'll work hard for your goal and you won't give up on the way. If this seems too hard for you, being goal oriented doesn't require you to be perfect. You're not going to always be positive and hard-working all of the time.

Even people who are already goal oriented do not act that way. They'll flatter, waver, and sometimes feel like giving up. But, in the end, they stick with what they've started with.

Always exercise regularly. Even when you don't necessarily have to, if you have time to waste, go hit the gym and give yourself a good workout.

You'll feel refreshed afterwards if you do. It's going to be an easy way to help you maintain your weight.

You should also make an effort to keep your goals. Alter them around a bit if you're starting to grow unmotivated. If whatever you're doing isn't necessarily working for you then try another plan.

You can always look back at what you're doing to see what worked best for you and what didn't. You don't have to always pick a plan that you have to work at with full effort. If a plan that you've made for yourself is requiring too much from you then change it up.

Even if you're the type to put in 100% effort of what you do, your efforts won't last for a very long time if you feel that you are forcing yourself to do it.

It's always good to look for people who would give you their support along the way. When you're trying to maintain your weight, it's always best to interact with those who share the same goals and mentality as you do.

It's going to make your efforts easier and you'll have a buddy that will do what you do. So if you have been craving for a friend to go work out at the gym with you then you're going to have a better time working out once you've find someone.

There isn't a limit as to who can support you. It can even be someone you don't even know. That might seem strange but you'll probably end up making a new friend by the time you realize it.

Meal Plans

Finally, we're going to talk about the types of foods that you should look for and the types of foods that you should stay away from.

As I've stated, when considering weight loss the kitchen is your best weapon. Your whole eating habits rely on the types of foods that are hidden in your kitchen. Whether you deny it or not, anything that is within your kitchen is going to get eaten. Even if you resist, you will eventually eat it.

The easiest way for you to resist the temptations is for you to throw away all of the unhealthy foods that you currently possess. Those unhealthy foods are stopping you from losing weight.

You should only be keeping healthy foods in your kitchen unless if they're expired. Make sure that all your healthy foods are kept up to date or else your stomach isn't going to have a very fun time digesting them.

I know it's going to be hard. The most common problem that people have is that they can't throw away food. One is because you've paid for it and it's yours to eat.

The second is that it'll be a waste of food if you were just to throw it away since there are other starving kids out there in the world. So, comeback for number one: since you've paid for it then you can give it away as a gift or share it with people you know.

Comeback for number two: why not give your food to the starving kids instead of trying to eat it to fill yourself up when you can replace it for healthy foods? The reason why you're having a hard time throwing away food is because you aren't making good enough reasons for you to throw them away.

If you're going to think about why you shouldn't then you should think about why you should. You're going to make a huge mistake if you think that you can slowly eat all of the junk food that you have without expecting any weight change. Throw it away. You can do it dramatically. It doesn't matter. Just do it. No exceptions.

If you can't manage to throw away food from your house, you're going to have a hard time managing when you're outside. It's a lot worse when you're out in public. There are a million things that go against you when you're outside.

You can practically find a fast food restaurant in every block and in every corner. This is when your kitchen would be the safest place for your stomach to be at. When you go outside, you need to develop a strong self-control for junk food. It might not come to you immediately, but it'll come over time.

The difference between being outside and being inside your house is that, when you're inside, it doesn't take willpower to avoid unhealthy foods. As long as your kitchen doesn't have any junk left inside of it then you're good to go.

Other People

If you're not living alone then the people living with you become a factor in your eating habits. This is because, most of the time, they won't try to eat healthy like you do. It's rare for anyone to abandon their usual food style in order to match with someone else's.

Your roommates and parents are going to be the majority. If you still live with your parents then the best way is for you to ask them to compromise with you. Have them put their junk food away from plain sight so it doesn't tempt you in any way. If your parents like to pull pranks on you then think of it as a sign that they are trying to improve your willpower. Other than that, make sure that your foods are easily seen compared to their junk foods.

If you both share the fridge, put their food in the back so the first thing that you would see when you open the fridge is your food which should be healthy foods. If anything, you can even buy your own fridge and keep it in your room so you won't have to go out into the kitchen to pick up food all of the time.

Also, if you know where they keep their foods then be sure to avoid those places. Temptation is right around the corner and behind closed doors.

The same would apply to your spouse, girlfriend or boyfriend. This should be a little easier than compromising with your parents because your partner doesn't necessarily dominate over you. You can always ask your partner to hide their food somewhere else. If they disagree then you can be mean about it if you want to. You can always throw away their food when they aren't around and make up some excuse so that they'll start hiding their foods away from you. Be careful though. You have to be very shady when you do this otherwise they will be furious at you.

Also, when you're throwing their food down the trash, bury it deep in there so they can't see it. If, in the case where you're really craving it because you can't defy the temptation then you can eat some. Just make sure that you don't overdo it.

Be sure to burn off some calories before you eat any type of junk food. This way, it'll stop you from giving in all the time. The more inconvenient it is for you to eat junk food the more you'll stay away from them.

If you're married and have kids then it shouldn't be much of a problem. They are your kids. In your house and under your roof, your word is and should be law.

It's your responsibility to make sure that they are eating healthy foods, especially if the money that is funding them is coming out of your paycheck. Of course, they are going to whine and complain and possibly cry, but, in the end, what can they do.

They're kids. They are going to find ways to make you want to spoil them. When this happens you have to be strong. Don't allow your kids to take over you. As a parent, you would know what's best.

Food to Toss

These are some of the types of foods that you should consider throwing away when you're emptying your fridge.

1. Frozen Meals

Frozen meals aren't at all healthy. Yea it's easy to make and everything since all you have to do is to heat it up. However, it doesn't necessarily help you in any way but to make you gain weight. You might not have known this but frozen meals are high processed foods and they're laden with sodium. These types of foods will often trigger your hunger and cravings because of the high sodium intake. Not to mention that those foods are completely tasteless.

Ice-cream and other frozen deserts should be tossed out too. Nowadays, you can find low-fat ice-cream almost anywhere. Unfortunately, just because the name says low-fat in it doesn't mean that it is. I've mentioned this before, low-fat foods will only make you fatter.

For ice-creams they are filled with sugar, artificial flavors, factory-created fats, colorings, chemicals, and preservatives. Meaning that not only is it fattening but it's also unhealthy. That doesn't mean that you are completely banned from eating ice-cream. It just means that you shouldn't eat so much. If you're planning on eating ice-cream, chose the most inconvenient method for you to get some. Buy it from a store rather than a whole carton.

2. Bread

This might seem weird to you since bread is usually considered as healthy foods. However, that doesn't mean that bread can't be factory made either. Unless if the bread is whole-bread, you shouldn't eat them all of the time. It's going to be like eating sugar.

3. Fridge

There are a lot of foods that can be placed in the fridge. Sometimes, if you're unsure of whether or not the food is unhealthy, check the food label. Obviously, if there are ingredients that you can barely pronounce or that it has a lot of sugar, it's going to be a junk food.

The types of foods that you want to look for are whole foods. Unless processed junk food, whole foods don't last for a very long time at room temperature which means that you would have to eat them within a short amount of time.

Yogurt is often placed in the fridge also. The flavored yogurts already carry loads of extra sugar and calories to begin with. If you're planning on eating yogurt then you just eat the plain ones.

If you want to have flavored yogurt then you should mix in your own fresh fruits in there. It's healthier and will taste a lot better than the already flavored yogurt that is filled with twice the sugar.

Get rid of any flavored drinks as well as sodas and fruit juice.

They are also filled with sugar and are completely unhealthy for you. We all know how bad it is for us to drink sodas but we still do it anyways. Well, when you're trying to lose weight, stop drinking them. Don't drink flavored drinks and fruit juice either.

Fruit juice isn't even healthy for you. If you want fruit juice you should just make it yourself. It might take a bit more effort but it's a lot healthier since you're using fresh fruits. For beverages, your best choice would be water or green tea. You can never go wrong with water.

4. Dressings

Dressings are dressings. They are mainly used as an additional taste for food but it's not as if they're harmless. For the light dressings, they may carry less fat and calories compared to the original dressings but they are filled with sugar or high fructose corn syrup. Regular dressings are filled with fats and calories. Either way, both are bad to eat.

5. Other Foods

Throw away all types of chips. It doesn't matter how healthy the bag seems to be, chips are chips. They are unhealthy and should be rid of. Cookies and crackers also need to go.

Don't bother thinking about keeping the low fat ones. If it's unhealthy to begin with, it's going to be unhealthy no matter what you do to it. All baking ingredients should go too. If you pay attention to the package labels on those things then you should know that those ingredients are all chemically made.

I've already stated that bread should be tossed out too unless if they are 100% whole wheat. The same applies to pasta. Unless if it's 100% whole wheat it needs to go. Don't bother asking about canned food. It's pretty obvious as to how unhealthy those cans are.

Eating Rules

Did you know that one pound of fat tissue contains about 3,500 calories? So that means that in order for you to lose about 2 pounds per week you would need to lose about 7,500 calories in total. Even if it seems a lot to lose, it's possible.

If you were to eat about 1,600 calories per day then you would be able to lose about 1-2 pounds per week. For most people, however, they would need more or they would need less. This would also depend on how your body works.

If you're the active type who constantly exercises on a daily basis then you would probably go past the 1,600 calories per day amount. In doing so you would double the portion of your snacks. If you're the type that would need less than 1,600 calories per day because you aren't as active then you should leave some food leftover.

In the case if you were to go over the 16,000 calories limit then you would be adding more weight to yourself because your body isn't able to burn that amount of calories at the rate that it's supposed to. Watch how your body works before changing your calorie consumption.

There are a couple of eating rules that you should keep in mind during the weight loss program. It's going to help make weight loss seem a lot easier than what you would think it would be.

1. Budget Calories

I've mentioned this before: keep track of what you eat per day. Remember, for an average person you would eat around 1,600 calories per day in order to lose the minimum amount of weight each week.

Always keep in mind of what you're eating and how many calories it contains. Of course, it won't always be on your mind since you'll have better things to think about but always be aware of it. Just remember that any excessive calories that you feed to your body will turn into fat.

The easiest approach is to keep processed foods and liquid calories down to a minimum and replace them with whole foods. This way, not only will you get enough for your money but you'll be eating food that has the lowest calorie density and the highest nutritional content and potential to fill you up.

2. Protein

Make sure that you buy food that provides you with enough protein for the day. Protein is vital since it keeps you from losing muscles and it also makes you fuller as it decreases your appetite.

In addition, it provides slow energy release that helps keep your blood sugar levels stable. Nevertheless, you should be careful as to how many grams of protein you are consuming for the day. A good amount per day would be 0.9 grams per pound of your target bodyweight.

So, basically, whatever weight that you are striving to achieve for you would multiply that weight with 0.9. Your answer would be the amount of protein that you would consume for the day.

3. Vegetables

If you're a vegetable hater then you have to start liking them. Vegetables are very good to eat when you're trying to lose weight. This is because vegetables provide a lot of nutrients and fiber, yet fewer calories.

It's recommended that you should get about 5-6 servings of non starchy vegetables per day. If you absolutely cannot stand eating vegetables, look up recipes on how you can make them suited to your taste. Think vegetarian.

4. Fats

Fats are actually good for you, believe it or not. A good 30% of your diet should come from fat. Even if you were told that fats were bad there are good fats and bad fats. The bad fats are saturated fat and trans fat. These are the type of fats that you would want to avoid the most. Even if you don't approve of this you have to eat fat anyways. Fats provide tastes to your meals which is why low-fat foods are tasteless.

5. Fruits

Fruits have the same standing as vegetables only that should eat about 2-3 fruits per day. It's better than eating sweet junk food all of the time. Fruits are both sweet and delicious and it adds a good amount of fiber that can fill you up without you having to worry about consuming too much calories.

In addition to that, you can also make smoothies and slushiest from fresh fruits. It's cheaper and healthier.

6. Test

This is the part where you have to be sure that whatever you're eating is healthy. More or less, it's a natural test. You have to check to see if the food that you're planning to eat passes the natural test. By natural I mean actual food that aren't produced and altered through chemical means. These are the type of foods that you can find in nature with barely any changes done to it.

It's very easy to tell whether a food has passed the natural test. Processed foods usually come in colorful containers, bags, boxes, jars, or wrappers.

Basically anything that looks nice and attracts your attention. Another way is to look at the food labels. If it's processed you won't be able to pronounce the words let alone know what type of ingredient it is.

If an ingredient sounds scientific then it's been chemically produced. For whole foods, their ingredients would only range up to three and the food looks a lot less packaged.

7. Eat

The whole purpose of losing weight is to eat so you can lose weight. That might not have made any sense but it that's the way our bodies work so it can't be helped.

You don't want to go on for more than 4 hours without eating any type of food. Any type of liquids that you can feel full from does not count. Going too long a period without having any food in your belly would make you risk not being able to think properly.

From that hunger, you won't be able to make proper food choices. You'll most likely end up picking out a quick snack that is high on calories in order for you to fill yourself up in a short amount of time.

You're also most likely going to eat too quickly and your stomach won't be able to digest it all at once which will cause you to want seconds.

8. Percent Rule

In weight loss, you are not required to put in your 100% effort. In fact, if weight loss actually did require people to put in their whole effort then most people would have a much harder time trying to continue to lose weight.

The beauty of weight loss is that you don't have to put in all of your efforts to succeed. You would still need effort but only at 90% rather than 100%. Discipline is good but too much will cause you to lose motivation.

With only 90% effort, you can still have some of your favorite treats as long as you don't take it in big increments and that you're not eating it every single day. Once in a while is fine but even if you do eat it once in a while, keep the portion size down to a minimum.

Your remaining 10% effort will be for you to eat whatever you want, but be careful not let that percentage rise higher than 10.

It might be that 10% is too little for your own freedom of food choice but that's because the remaining 90% requires you to know how to maintain your responsibilities so you won't fall off track.

Shopping

If you're the type who's a conservative spender then you'll have an easier time shopping than others. When people often walk into a store they'll buy something on the spot simply because they crave it or it's on sale.

Conservative spenders are the type of people who only buys what they need or what they planned to buy. Not many people are conservative spenders since there's always temptations around every corner.

Even in grocery stores there are temptations, especially the junk foods that they have. There are sales, discounts, and deals lay out in big bold letters for you, especially in the junk aisle.

If you're easily tempted by food then the best way is for you to stay along the perimeter of the store. Most stores keep their healthy foods in the outer sections while the junk food and other stuff are kept in the inner section.

Even when there is a food that states how healthy it is for you, always look at the food labels. If it doesn't pass the natural test then it's obviously unhealthy.

When buying packaged foods, look for both the serving size and the number of servings there is in total. You would need to do basic math when you're looking at this. If there is another product that is similar to what you're buying, compare them.

Pick the product that has the least amount of calories and is healthy for you. Always look at the fat and sugar per servings since those are also important.

Look for low-sodium foods and foods that are low in Trans and saturated fat. Avoid Trans fat as much as you can as well as any other product with too much ingredients listed.

Keep in mind that shopping for healthy food in a healthy food store does not mean that you're buying healthy food. Food companies have ways to make their food products seem healthy but they can't lie about what's in it. So take that up to your advantage and use it. Don't bother looking for bargains.

When you're on a diet, what matters is how healthy your food is not how cheap a price you can get it for. Money comes after health. If you're really craving junk food then buy a small pack so you don't end up eating too much.

It's always good to shop from a grocery list. It's actually one of the best method since you already know what you want to buy.

Having a list will help you finish your shopping faster and it'll stop you from buying unnecessary foods. You'll be able to save time and money.

Always stay true to the same store. When you're grocery shopping it's best if you don't move around so much. This is because, if you shop at the exact same store for a long time, you would already know where everything is placed at. Thus, it further shortens the time that you would spend there. When you go to a new store you wouldn't know where everything is placed at so you would spend more time searching around for what you want.

As you're looking around, you could be distracted with other food products that the store has. Eventually, you're going to keep adding unnecessary foods to your cart even if you don't need to.

Work yourself. Don't buy so much food that will help you last for more than a month. Only buy foods that will last you for a week. This is so you can resupply once every week. The reason why I'm saying this is to get you to exercise. Pick a store near your house and walk there.

By doing so you'll be burning calories by walking to and from the store and it'll stop you from hauling back too many heavy foods. Remember to always have a fridge filled with food. If there's nothing to eat then you'll grow hungry and will start to eat junk food.

When you go to do your grocery shopping, pick a day that you know there's not going to be so many people. If the store is almost empty then it's easier for you to finish since there isn't a lot of people waiting in line.

If the day is full then you're most likely going to wander around to kill time.

Cooking

Unless if you actually like going through the effort of cooking your meals then cooking is going to come off as a pain to you. This is why I am providing you with a few methods to simplify your cooking life for you.

1. Vegetables

When you buy vegetables, chop them up and put them in food storage containers as soon as you get home. This way, you won't have to bother yourself by cutting them up when you actually want to cook with those ingredients. It'll be ready and chopped up for your convenience. All you have to do is rinse them again to make sure that the veggies are clean and are ready to cook. This will save you a lot of time, especially if you're lazy that day.

2. Salsa

If you want an additional flavor or dressing, add salsa. Salsa is the key to everything. Why? Because it's low in calories and high in nutrients. Best of all, salsa goes with everything.

It's good, healthy, and easy to make. You don't even have to buy salsa. It'll probably taste better if you just make it yourself since you have more control over what ingredients you want in there.

3. Portions

Whenever you cook your meals, make enough so that it'll be able to last for a couple of days. If you don't like to cook or you're a busy person then I highly recommend you do this. You can either double or triple the portion size of your food when you make it and whatever you don't eat can be used as leftovers for the next couple of days.

Make sure that you don't eat a lot just because you've made a lot. The point of cooking ahead is to save time, not to fatten you up.

The best day to cook ahead would be Sunday only because it's usually a lazy day. Most people do not work on Sunday so they have the whole day to do whatever the want. Use this day to cook ahead. Otherwise, you're going to be forcing yourself to cook later on.

Obstacles

Even when you have your plans laid out for you it's still hard to keep up with it all of the time. There are many other obstacles that you have to face when you're on the diet plan.

Your kitchen is only the first step. The second step is for you to know what to do when you're invited to go eat outside or when you're invited to a party.

When you're eating out you should keep in mind that no matter how healthy or how less the food may seem, it's going to pack a bunch of calories. So what do you do to avoid consuming too much calories in one meal?

First, it's always best to go out to eat on a day where you know that you will feel stressed out and tired. This would be the day where you are too lazy to cook anything to eat. When you eat out, eat before the time that you would normally eat. This would give your body more time to digest the food once you've eaten it.

Decide on what kind of food you want to eat before you leave the house. It'll help narrow down your choices and it'll keep you from eating any excessive foods. It'll also make it easier for you to research the amount of calories those types of foods will carry.

Secondly, when you're eating outside food, don't eat until you are completely full. Eat until you are 80% full. If you don't know what that feeling is like then it's basically when you know that you can stop eating but your body can eat more.

Whatever it is that you don't finish can be saved as leftovers for your next meal. If anything, eat something before you leave so you won't order a large portion when you arrive.

Thirdly, drink lots of water. You can never go wrong with water. Plus, when you drink water as you're eating you will start to feel full before you're able to finish your meal.

In the situation where you're allowed to drink alcohol when you're out because you have a fixed ride home, don't drink it. I recommend that you don't look at the menu for alcohol. If you feel that you must have it because you can't hold back anymore then have it during the meal and not before or after it.

Fourthly, eat slowly. You can pretend that it's your last meal of the day and that you won't be able to eat anything else afterwards until the next day. That or you can pretend that it's your last meal, period. Savor the food and slowly chew it. If you eat slowly, you'll be able to taste the fullness better.

Conclusion

Overall, when approaching weight loss, you should keep in mind that it's not going to be very easy, but it's not going to be very hard either. The easier you make it on yourself the easier it'll be for you to succeed.

Don't forget that exercise is everything. The most important factor of weight loss is eating. Don't forget that the kitchen is your best friend. You don't have to give your 100% effort in order to succeed.

A good rate is 90%. Don't forget that if you break away from the diet plan for one day it doesn't mean that you should break it for the rest of the day. You should immediately follow back into your plan.

Don't make excuses for not continuing what you started. You can make an excuse every single day for the rest of your life but you won't get very far if you do. Don't make it harder on yourself.

Simplicity is key.

www.ingramcontent.com/pod-product-compliance
Lightning Source LLC
Chambersburg PA
CBHW020351290526
45785CB00005B/2227